OUTLIVE YOUR LONGEVITY

ROBERTS R. WESTON

COPYRIGHT MESSAGE

TABLE OF CONTENT

INTRODUCTION

In a quiet suburban neighborhood, Mr. Edward Morrison, seventy-eight, lived a solitary life after his wife's passing. A retired mechanic, Edward prided himself on his independence and resilience. Yet, over the years, he ignored signs of declining health—a persistent cough, joint pain, and occasional dizziness.

One scorching summer day, while tinkering under a car hood, a sudden wave of dizziness gripped Edward. Gasping for air, he collapsed to the ground, clutching his chest. A neighbor, Mrs. Harris, rushed to his aid upon seeing him from across the street.

"Edward! What happened?" Mrs. Harris cried out in alarm.

Struggling to speak, Edward managed, "Chest… pain… can't breathe…"

Mrs. Harris immediately called 911. Paramedics arrived swiftly, recognizing signs of a severe heart attack exacerbated by untreated hypertension and cardiovascular strain. Edward was rushed to the hospital, drifting in and out of consciousness.

In the emergency room, doctors worked urgently to stabilize Edward. His heart had suffered extensive damage from years of neglecting high blood pressure and underlying cardiac issues. Emergency procedures followed, but the road to recovery was uncertain.

Days passed in the hospital, Edward's weakened body fighting against the aftermath of his neglect. His children, summoned by urgency, gathered at his bedside, grappling with the realization of his fragile state.

Edward's recovery was slow and fraught with complications. Physical therapy sessions aimed to rebuild his strength, while nurses monitored his progress vigilantly. Each day brought small victories and setbacks, highlighting Edward's resilience amid regret.

Reflecting from his hospital bed, Edward grasped the consequences of his choices—decades of hard work overshadowed by the weight of neglect. Discharged eventually, he returned to a home that felt emptier, the workshop where he once found solace was now a reminder of his mortality.

With support from his children and neighbors, Edward committed to regular medical appointments, medication adherence, and a healthier lifestyle. Months passed, and his strength gradually returned. He found solace in simple pleasures, morning coffee on the porch, laughter of grandchildren during visits, and moments of quiet reflection.

Yet, scars of neglect remained, etched in his weathered face and weary bones. Edward understood now that time was precious, and not to be taken for granted. Watching sunsets cast golden hues over the suburban neighborhood, he vowed to cherish each moment and embrace his second chance to live fully and appreciate life's fragile beauty.

Aging is an inevitable journey we all embark on from the moment we are born. It is a process that occurs throughout our entire lives and is characterized by changes in our physical, mental, and social environments. Aging is also a time of growth, wisdom, and transformation, despite the fact that it is typically viewed through the lens of decline and loss. This book will discuss ways to embrace and thrive in this phase of life, as well as the many facets of aging and its challenges and opportunities.

Understanding aging, a multi-dimensional process

Social, psychological, and biological factors all play a role in aging. From a biological point of view, it involves gradual changes in the systems of our body, such as a decrease in muscle mass, bone density, sensory perception, and organ function. Both an increase in disease susceptibility and a decrease in physical resilience may result from these changes. Alterations in cognition, memory, and emotional regulation can occur psychologically with aging. While some cognitive abilities may decline as we get older, others, like wisdom and emotional intelligence, frequently continue to grow and become more sophisticated. Alterations in personality traits and priorities may occur in older adults, as well as an increased sense of resilience and acceptance. Roles and relationships shift as people age socially. A person's sense of identity and well-being can be affected by changes in social networks, retirement, and the death of loved ones. Volunteering, mentoring, and participating in community activities, on the other hand, frequently provide older adults with new avenues of fulfillment.

Aging Challenges
Aging presents numerous challenges despite its inherent richness. Health is one of the main concerns. As we get older, the prevalence of chronic conditions like arthritis, diabetes, cardiovascular diseases, and dementia rises, necessitating careful management and adaptation.

Another vital aspect is mental health. Older adults may experience depression and anxiety, which is frequently exacerbated by factors such as social isolation, financial stress, or the loss of independence. For the sake of overall health, it is essential to address mental health needs. Many older people, especially those who are retiring and relying on fixed incomes, are particularly concerned about their financial security. To maintain financial stability and tranquility, it is essential to plan for retirement, manage savings, and navigate healthcare costs.

Last but not least, issues can arise as a result of how society views aging. Ageism, or age-based discrimination, can result in stereotypes, prejudice, and fewer opportunities for older people. Promoting inclusivity, challenging stereotypes, and advocating for policies that support older adults are all necessary for overcoming ageist attitudes.

Taking Advantage of Opportunities:

Aging presents a wealth of opportunities for development, fulfillment, and contribution in spite of the challenges. The following are some strategies for embracing and maximizing later life:

Physical Well-Being:
Maintaining mobility and physical health requires regular exercise, a healthy diet, and preventative healthcare. Strength, flexibility, and overall well-being can all be improved through activities like yoga, swimming, or walking.

Mental and Emotional Well-Being:
Do things like solve puzzles, read, or learn new skills that make your brain work harder. Stress can be reduced and emotional resilience enhanced by practicing mindfulness and relaxation techniques.

Social Connections
Make meaningful connections with friends, family, and members of the community. Participate in clubs, volunteer work, or interest groups to maintain social activity. Support, companionship, and a sense of belonging can be gained by maintaining a robust social network.

Lifelong Learning:
Engage in hobbies, courses, or lectures to maintain intellectual curiosity and curiosity. Lifelong learning not only keeps the mind sharp, but also helps people grow and feel fulfilled. Purpose and Meaning: Look for activities that give your life purpose and meaning, like mentoring others, pursuing your creative interests, or advocating for causes you care about. In later life, having a sense of purpose can improve overall well-being and satisfaction.

Adaptability:
Resilience and adaptability in the face of change are essential. Life transitions like health issues or retirement may necessitate adjustments, but they also present chances for personal development and exploration.

CHAPTER ONE

UNDERSTANDING THE SCIENCE OF AGING

Aging is as much a part of human life as infancy, childhood, and adolescence and begins as soon as one reaches adulthood. The changes that take place between a person's maturity and death are the primary focus of the field of gerontology, the study of aging. The identification of the factors that influence these changes is the objective of research in gerontology. Putting this knowledge to use can lessen the severity of some disabilities that come with aging.

Aging does not happen overnight. Instead, it is an ongoing biological process that follows us from the moment we are born until the moment we die. The human lifespan has nearly doubled in the last 120 years as a result of the advancement of medical techniques and hygiene practices. The negative aspect of this optimistic scenario is that age-related diseases will affect an increasing number of people. Every living thing gets older. But why do we need to get older? Does one have a "biological sense"? Experts are still debating the best way to respond to these questions. Internal and external factors both play a significant role in aging, according to a number of insights and theories. The following are some of the most frequently raised theories in aging research.

AGING ON A BIOLOGICAL LEVEL

The fundamental biological factors that contribute to aging as well as the general state of health care included in the biological physiological aspects of aging.

It is evident that the individual must undergo changes that increase his or her susceptibility to disease, as the likelihood of death increases rapidly with age. A young adult might recover from pneumonia quickly, but an elderly person might die. Many organs, including the heart, kidneys, brain, and lungs, show a gradual decline over time, according to physiologists.

The individual's reserve capacities are reduced as a result of the loss of cells from these organs, which accounts for a portion of this decline. Additionally, the elderly person's remaining cells may not perform as well as those of the young. Because some cellular enzymes may be less active, chemical reactions may take longer to complete. The cell might eventually die.

HOW OUR HEART AGE

Two sides make up the heart. In order to eliminate carbon dioxide and deliver oxygen to the lungs, the right side pumps blood. The body receives oxygen-rich blood from the left side. The aorta and the arteries, which branch out and become ever-smaller as they enter the tissues, carry blood out of the heart. They develop into tiny capillaries within the tissues. The blood passes through capillaries to deliver oxygen and nutrients to the tissues and to receive carbon dioxide and wastes from the tissues. After that, the vessels begin to congregate into ever-larger veins that carry blood back to the heart.

The natural pacemaker system in the heart regulates the heartbeat. Fibrous tissue and fat deposits may form along this system's pathways. Some of the cells in the natural pacemaker, the sinoatrial or SA node, die. The heart rate might slow down a little as a result of these changes. Some people experience a slight increase in heart size, particularly in the left ventricle. Despite the overall larger heart, the chamber's capacity to hold blood may actually decrease as the heart wall thickens. It might fill more slowly. A normal healthy older person's electro cardiogram (ECG) frequently differs slightly from that of a healthy younger adult due to heart changes. Arrhythmias, or abnormal rhythms, like atrial fibrillation, are more prevalent in older people. They can be brought on by a variety of heart diseases. Deposits of lipofuscin, also known as the "aging pigment," are part of normal heart changes. The cells of the heart muscle degenerate slightly. The thickening and stiffening of the heart's valves, which direct blood flow, is a normal part of aging. Valve stiffness is a common cause of heart murmurs in older people.

DISEASES AFFECTING THE HEART

Heart disease refers to any problem affecting the heart, such as coronary artery disease, and heart failure.

According to the Centers for Disease Control and Prevention (CDC), heart disease is the leading cause of death in the United States. Around 1 in 4 deathsTrusted Source in the U.S. occur due to heart disease, and the condition affects all genders as well as all racial and ethnic groups.

Some of these diseases are:

CORONARY ARTERY DISEASE

The most prevalent form of heart disease is coronary artery disease, also known as coronary heart disease. It occurs when plaque builds up in the arteries that carry blood to the heart. They harden and narrow as a result. Cholesterol and other substances are present in plaque. As a result, the heart receives less oxygen and nutrients from the blood supply. The heart muscle weakens over time, increasing the likelihood of heart failure and arrhythmias. Atherosclerosis refers to the condition in which plaque builds up in the arteries. A heart attack can result from blockages in the arteries breaking apart and stopping blood flow.

HEART ARRHYTHMIA

Your heart's rhythm is erratic when you have an arrhythmia. Serious arrhythmias can occur on their own or as a result of other heart conditions.

HEART VALVE DISEASE

The four valves in your heart open and close to direct blood flow between the lungs, blood vessels, and the heart's four chambers. A valve may struggle to open and close correctly due to an abnormality. Blood may leak or your blood flow may become restricted as a result. It's possible that your valve doesn't work right when it opens and closes. Heart valve issues can be brought on by an infection like rheumatoid arthritis, congenital heart disease, high blood pressure, coronary artery disease, or a heart attack.

HOW OUR BRAIN AGE

The brain creates more than a million new neural connections every second during the early years of life. The brain grows to approximately 90% of its adult volume by the age of six. The brain then begins to shrink in our 30s and 40s with an even greater rate of shrinkage by the age of 60. The appearance of the brain begins to change in the same way that wrinkles and gray hair begin to appear later in life. Additionally, the physical morphing of our brains will alter our cognitive abilities. We typically experience the following changes as we get older:

Brain mass:
Although the total volume of the brain decreases with age, the frontal lobe and the hippocampus, which are particular regions of the brain that are responsible for cognitive functions, shrink more than other regions. Behind the forehead, you'll find the frontal lobes. They are thought to be the centers of human behavior and emotional control for our personalities. They are the largest lobes

in the human brain. The hippocampus is a complex structure in the temporal lobe of the brain. It has a significant impact on memory and learning. The hippocampus is susceptible to a wide range of mental and neurological conditions, according to research.

Cortical density

The thinning of the brain's outer corrugated surface as a result of fewer synaptic connections is referred to as cortical density. Age also thins our cerebral cortex, the wrinkled outer layer of the brain that contains the bodies of neuronal cells. The frontal lobes and a portion of the temporal lobe are particularly affected by cortical thinning, which occurs in a pattern similar to that of volume loss. A decrease in density results in fewer connections, which may slow down cognitive processing.

White matter:

White matter is made up of myelinated nerve fibers that are bundled into tracts and transmit nerve signals between brain cells. Myelin shrinks, according to researchers, as we get older, stymieing processing and impairing cognitive function. White matter is a vast network of neural connections that connects the limbic system, the brain's emotion center, to all four of the brain's lobes (frontal, temporal, parietal, and occipital).

Neurotransmitters:

The brain begins to produce various levels of chemicals that affect the production of neurotransmitters and proteins, eventually leading to cognitive decline. Older people may experience memory problems like having trouble remembering names or words, losing focus, or being unable to do more than one thing at a time. Neurons begin to die and cells also produce a compound called amyloid-beta as the brain ages. Amyloid beta is typically linked to Alzheimer's disease. It can also be found in the aging brain of a person. The presence of amyloid-beta plaques, or prions, in the brain may indicate Alzheimer's disease. Additionally, it may be a sign of normal aging when there are plaque signs but no prions.

In general, taking care of oneself becomes more challenging for older people as the brain ages.

HOW THE SKIN AGE

Environmental factors, genetics, nutrition, and other factors all play a role in skin changes. However, exposure to the sun is the single most important factor. This can be seen by contrasting sun-protected areas of your body with those that are regularly exposed to the sun. Sun damage seems to be mitigated in some way by natural pigments. People with fair skin and blue eyes have more changes in their skin as they get older than people with darker skin that has more pigment.

Changes with age

Despite the same number of cell layers, aging thins the epidermis, or outer skin layer. Melanocytes, or cells that contain pigment, decrease in number. The size of the remaining melanocytes grows. Skin that is getting older appears thinner, paler, and transparent. Sun-exposed areas may develop age spots, also known as "liver spots." Lentigos is the medical term for these areas. The skin loses its elasticity and strength as a result of changes in the connective tissue. Elastosis is the term for this. Solar elastosis makes it more obvious in areas that are exposed to the sun. The leathery, weather-worn appearance that farmers, sailors, and other people who spend a lot of time outside get from elastosis is common. The dermis's blood vessels become more fragile. Cherry angiomas, under-the-skin bleeding (commonly referred to as senile purpura), and bruising are the results of this. As we get older, our sebaceous glands produce less oil. After the age of 80, men experience a slight decline. After menopause, women produce less oil over time. The skin may become dry and irritated as a result of this, making it harder to keep it moist. There is less padding and insulation in the subcutaneous fat layer as it thins. As a result, you are less able to regulate your body temperature and run the risk of sustaining skin injuries. In cold weather, you run the risk of becoming hypothermic because you have less natural insulation. The fat layer absorbs some medicines. This layer's shrinkage may alter how these medicines work. Less sweat is produced by the sweat glands. It's harder to keep cool because of this. Your chance of getting heat stroke or overheating goes up. Older people are more likely to have skin tags, warts, brown rough patches (seborrheic keratoses), and other bumps. Pinkish rough patches, also known as actinic keratosis, are also common and have a small chance of developing into skin cancer. Additionally, skin cancers are frequently found in sun-exposed locations.

(We would have go on and on, but advancing would mean we are going beyond the scope and aim of this book.
To know more about biological age-related problems please consult your physician).

AGING ON A MENTAL LEVEL
A greater focus on the psychological aspects of aging has resulted from an increase in the number of older people and an increase in life

expectancy worldwide. A growing body of evidence suggests that successful aging is multifaceted, including a level of psychological, physical, and social well-being. As populations age, geropsychology is becoming more and more important. The field of geropsychology focuses on comprehending, treating, and enhancing the mental health of older adults. It's possible that many older adults with mental health issues are not getting the right treatment at the moment. It is essential to promptly identify and treat mental health issues in older adults. Medicines and psychosocial interventions are suggested.

Mental health and psychological changes
Mental health and well-being are just as important as ever when someone is older. In this age group, mental and neurological disorders account for 6.6% of the total disability. A mental illness affects about 15% of adults over the age of 60.
In addition to physical changes, aging can have a number of psychological effects on your life that can lower its quality. Psychological effects can

begin before you even notice the first visible signs of aging. Because it affects their social and professional lives, both men and women become more self-conscious about their appearance and body shape. Anxiety, mild to moderate depression, and increased distress may result from this. One of the most common side effects of getting older is depression. It's not always caused by getting older; rather, it's caused by personal and social factors. As their features deteriorate over time, overly concerned individuals may experience depression. This condition can also be brought on by a lack of social interaction or being abandoned by friends or family. Your mental health deteriorates over time on a general scale. The weakening of your nervous system could also be the cause of this. Conditions such as delirium, dementia, stroke, Alzheimer's disease, schizophrenia, and others are more likely. A person's intelligence and memory capacity may also be affected. In general, these conditions are frequently multifactorial and brought on by a variety of other aging-related factors.

Sadly, mental illness is underdiagnosed among seniors, and many mental health issues are treated ineffectively. Additionally, older adults are already at risk for suicide, and mental illness raises that risk even more. Although seniors make up 12% of the population, they account for 18% of suicides, which may surprise you. It is essential for all of us to be able to recognize the symptoms of mental illness in elderly people in order to assist them in receiving the assistance they require to alleviate their symptoms and enhance their quality of life.

Mental illness red flags includes

- Isolation

Depression or other mental health issues may be the cause of social withdrawal.

- Changes in appetite

An underlying mental health issue may be the cause of sudden weight loss or gain, appetite changes, or both.

- Confusion

Disorientation in the elderly can also be a sign of major depression or psychosis, despite the common misconception that it is a sign of dementia.

- Physical symptoms that don't make sense. Physical manifestations of mental health issues include muscle tension and pain, sweating and shivering, digestive issues, and changes in bowel habits.

- Feelings of hopelessness, worthlessness, or excessive guilt

Often, depression and other mood disorders cause people to feel worthless, empty, sad, or guilty in an inappropriate way. A common misconception is that depression is a normal part of getting older.

Although this is not true, there are a number of factors that increase an individual's risk of developing depression and other mental health disorders as they get older, such as the grief and loss of loved ones, chronic health conditions, or diminished functioning that frequently accompany aging. In a senior's life, the right diagnosis and treatment can make all the difference. Contact a mental health professional right away and ask for assistance if you or someone you care about is exhibiting symptoms of mental health issues.

AGING ON A SOCIAL LEVEL

Why is it important to people's lives if aging only causes relatively minor, universal, and inevitable changes to physical or cognitive functioning, personality structure, and adult development? The social meanings, structures, and procedures associated with age are the primary reasons why age is significant. The social world in which we live has defined gray hair, wrinkles, longer reaction times, and even some short-term memory loss as meaningful characteristics. Erroneous beliefs about the effects of aging on physical and mental capabilities are at the root of a lot of the social meaning attached to aging. We do not automatically become rigid in our thinking, forgetful, or incapable of engaging in our favorite physical or intellectual pursuits as we age. The majority of people view aging as a gradual process in which we make up for most of it and allow it to have little effect on our day-to-day lives. Age, on the other hand, is used by society to assign roles, move people into and out of positions within the social structure, allocate resources, and classify individuals. Utilizing age to allocate opportunities is a reasonable strategy in its most benevolent form. For instance, the minimum age for employment in our society is set. These laws were enacted to prevent young people from being exploited, and some argue that they are beneficial to the labor force because they control the flow of new workers into the workforce. Age, on the other hand, artificially and unevenly restricts people's opportunities in a more restrictive manner. Gray hair, wrinkles, and the chronological age of 65, which is the most common indicator of old age, have no effect on one's ability to think clearly or physically.

They do, notwithstanding, significantly affect social associations and open doors for people in the social universes of business, day-to-day life, and local area commitment. Our assessment of the person's age and what that person's age represents to us have a significant impact on whether we would seriously consider them as a job candidate or as an interesting social partner. Again, this is not because gray hair or being 65 is a sign of competence or incompetence, of a dull or brilliant personality, or even because visible aging is inherently unattractive or attractive. We make these judgments because our society has shaped the meaning of aging in specific, mostly negative ways.

In our wild youth days, we burned cigarettes, drank liquor and make-out. But as we continue to grow up we realize that we are beginning to lose interest in some of these acts. Mainly due to the burden and enormous responsibility of starting a family and being a good parent or example to our children. Many people call this act maturity. Though, they are right but reality behind this is that maturity comes with age. When we are young we use acts of violence like watching WWE, boxing and so many other physical sports, some of us even took it a step further by delivering pain on our fellow humans.

But as you age, you may see yourself reflecting on your past deeds and you will find it hilarious and embarrassing. You might be thinking about the catalogs of friends you keep at a point in your life compared with the little you have now. Mind you, social aging doesn't have to be related to age numbers simply because some of us matured and soliloquized about life more than others. You might find a forty-year-old giving better life advice than an eighty-year-old.

Aging socially is what makes us real adults, from your heavy metal days to your present cool jazz age, from your hangover nights to your peaceful solo night sleep and your wild adventures seeking past to you now finding seemingly better joy in staying behind the doors of your house.

Life and everything will change all around you and you will find yourself embracing it. Some people will try to resist but they are only doing more harm than good.

Simply let it go.

Because yesterday was a gift

Today is a present

And tomorrow is a treasure waiting to unfold.

How you deal with yourself aging socially will determine how you age biologically and mentally. If you decide to wake up each morning and decide to be grumpy about your mammoth age and life then don't be surprised when your doctor tell you that you are at a high risk of developing hypertension and other cardiac diseases or your doctor tells you that you are mentally ailing and you might even find yourself in the store looking for beauty or wrinkles reducing creams. But if you wake up with joy to accept the present of today, exercise on a daily routine and put a wide smile on your face you are only going to find yourself looking younger and more beautiful than ever before.
Aging on a biological level.
Aging on a mental level. And
Aging on a social level.
These are the three ways by which we age.
They are inevitable but we can mold them into a blessing by utilizing them properly.

CHAPTER TWO

ANTI-AGING EXERCISES

WHAT IS EXERCISE?

Physical activity that improves or maintains fitness and overall health is called exercise. It is performed in light of multiple factors, including weight reduction or support, to help develop and further develop strength, foster muscles and the cardiovascular framework, level up athletic abilities, improve health, or essentially for satisfaction. Many people prefer to exercise outside, where they can socialize, exercise in groups, and improve their mental and physical health.

As we work out, our heart and breathing rates increase, which increases the bloodstream as the body requires more oxygen and fuel to the functioning muscles At rest, about 20% of blood flow reaches working muscles; during maximal exercise with large muscle groups, like running or cycling, this percentage can rise to over 80%.

These increases will be much smaller if the exercise intensity is low to moderate, and they will tend to stabilize after a few minutes at the same intensity.

Exercise is not about developing attractive and admirable muscles but more about keeping fit and developing a healthy body.

Seniors, we don't have to bust our aging butt in the gym to exercise. Back in those days, I could do like a hundred reps at a go, but now I can barely make it up to twenty reps in just a single day. Though I know I am lazy I realize that I don't have to suffer from body aches to muscle tears for the sake of exercising, then I discovered an exercise routine that works well for me. And I would share some with you

CHAIR YOGA

Chair yoga is a low-impact exercise that helps seniors improve their muscle strength, mobility, balance, and flexibility—all important aspects of their health. When compared to more traditional styles of yoga, chair yoga places less stress on the bones, joints, and muscles. Chair yoga has also been shown to improve mental health in older adults, which is a bonus. Participants in chair yoga regularly experience better quality sleep, fewer cases of depression, and a general sense of well-being.

What safety measures should I take?
The careful idea of yoga permits you to zero in on how your body feels while playing out the activity while taking full breaths to keep up with the center. You ought to constantly be mindful of how the posture feels and perceive inconvenience and agony. After a few sessions, you can gradually increase the intensity if you move gently.
Here are some safety tips for chair yoga: Relax your joints by inhaling and exhaling while moving your body.
Sit upright and Place your ankle over your knee.
Maintain a flat footing on the ground.
Try not to strain, avoiding bouncing or jerking.
What are chair yoga's fundamental poses?
Mountain Stance
Side-to-side bend

Kneel hug
Cow/cat
Helicopter
Hamstring stretch
Gluteal stretch.

SQUATS

If you have any desire to remain youthful, do squats! Thus, you are figuring out the whole body - especially, the hamstrings, the hips, the glutes, and the quads. Thus, it likewise reinforces your body's center. These activities likewise help to work on your equilibrium and your degree of coordination. If that wasn't already enough, squats invert maturing by developing your bone thickness!

HIGH IMPACT MOVEMENT - While this is definitely not a specific activity, a sort of movement ought to be played out that is actual in nature. For this reason, it has made this rundown. While exploring how exercise turns around maturing, you will find that most experts suggest taking part in high-effect developments.

These incorporate hopping, strong venturing, and exaggerated movement, all in all. In the event that you verify that you perform high-impact movement consistently, your bones will increase in thickness.

WALKING

Walking is an extraordinary method for improving or keeping up with your general well-being. Only 30 minutes consistently can increment cardiovascular wellness, fortify bones, lessen overabundance of muscle and fat, and lift muscle power and perseverance.

It can likewise decrease your gamble of creating conditions like coronary illness, type 2 diabetes, osteoporosis and a few tumors.

Dissimilar to a few different types of activity, walking is free and requires no extraordinary hardware or preparation.

Active work doesn't need to be vivacious or accomplished for significant stretches to work on your well-being.

Walking has a low effect, requires negligible hardware, should be possible whenever of day and can be performed at your own speed. You can get out and stroll without agonizing over the dangers related to certain more incredible types of activity.

Walking is likewise an extraordinary type of active work for individuals who are overweight, old, or who haven't practiced in quite a while.

Walking for entertainment only and wellness isn't restricted to walking around yourself around nearby neighborhood roads. There are different clubs, scenes and methodologies you can use to make walking an agreeable and social piece of your way of life.

YOGA

India is the home of yoga, a spiritual and physical practice. It is available to amateurs, and a great many people can receive the well-being rewards of consistently rehearsing yoga. The goal of yoga poses is to make a connection between the breath and the body. Consistent yoga practice can improve a person's flexibility, strength, and balance, in addition to lowering stress levels. Numerous studies on the health benefits of yoga have been conducted, according to trusted sources.

Maintaining a healthy weight, quitting smoking, and reducing symptoms of menopause are potential health benefits. Many advanced yoga poses are suitable for beginners, despite the fact that some may appear intimidating. Yoga can be started by most people.

CYCLING

Cycling is a low-impact, healthy activity that can be enjoyed by people of all ages, from infants to seniors.

Additionally, it is inexpensive, enjoyable, and green. Riding to work or the shops is one of the most time-effective methods for consolidating standard activity with your regular daily schedule. An expected one billion individuals ride bikes consistently - for transport, diversion and game. Cycling for fitness and health A general improvement in your health can be achieved in as little as two to four hours per week. Cycling is: It has less of an impact than most other forms of exercise, resulting in fewer strains and injuries. Cycling is a good way to tone your muscles because you pedal through all the major muscle groups. Cycling is easy because, unlike some other sports, it doesn't require a lot of physical skill.

The majority of people are familiar with bike riding, and once you learn it, you never forget it. Stamina and strength are improved by cycling, which also improves aerobic fitness. As intense as you like: If you're recovering from an injury or illness, cycling can be started at a very low intensity and built up to a demanding physical workout. A fun way to get fit. Cycling is more likely to keep you cycling regularly than other physical activities that keep you indoors or require special times or locations because of the excitement and adventure of coasting down hills. Cycling is a time-saving mode of transportation because it replaces sedentary (sitting) time spent driving a car or taking public transportation like buses, trains, or trams with healthy exercise.

SWIMMING
Swimming Exercises for Beginners

Sustainability is one of the most important aspects of physical fitness. Fitting exercise into your schedule and achieving your health objectives is easier when you find activities you enjoy. It's important to keep your exercise routine varied; different types of workouts can help you change it up and gain momentum. Swimming is a low-impact, full-body activity that is great for people of all sizes and shapes. Swimming for exercise will assist you with lessening pressure, further developing muscle strength, and backing your heart's well-being.

Advantages of Swimming for Exercise

Because swimming is a low-impact activity, it is suitable for people with joint conditions like arthritis, multiple sclerosis, and osteoporosis. Additionally, the water's gentle resistance makes it a safe workout. According to a 2016 study, swimming regularly helped osteoarthritic patients. For three months, the participants swam for 45 minutes each day, three times per week. They observed an improvement in muscle strength and physical limitations as a result.

With swimming, they even saw a significant decrease in stiffness and joint pain.

BENEFITS OF SWIMMING
It strengthens the cardiovascular system.
It strengthens the cardiovascular system. The heart, lungs, and circulatory system are all involved in cardiovascular exercise or cardio. This kind of exercise will be included in a comprehensive workout routine that includes swimming, for example. According to one study, "swimmers had 53%, 50%, and 49% lower all-cause mortality risk than did men who were sedentary, walkers, or runners, respectively, after adjustment for age, body mass index, smoking status, alcohol intake, and family history of cardiovascular disease."

An alternate studyTrusted Source, from 2016, demonstrates that swimming can assist with bringing down circulatory strain. In this study, fifteen overweight adult males completed eight weeks of swimming training and four weeks of detraining.

It can be done by people of all ages and fitness levels.

A few sorts of activity might be trying for individuals who are different from it or who feel exceptionally ill-suited. Swimming, on the other hand, allows people to progress at their own pace and can appeal to people who have never exercised before. Swimming can be learned at a young age, and most pools have a section for beginners and swimmers who prefer to swim slowly.

It is gentle on the joints

Swimming does not put too much stress on joints. As a result, swimming might be a good exercise for someone who has arthritis or a joint injury because the water's buoyancy relieves stress on the weight-bearing joints.

It is beneficial for injured individuals. Exercising with a lot of force can be difficult for someone with arthritis or another injury. Individuals who can't participate in high-effect, high-obstruction activities might lean toward swimming on the grounds that the water delicately upholds the muscles.

Strengthens your heart

Need to keep your ticker at top capability? One of the keys to a healthy heart is cardiovascular exercise, and swimming has clear benefits for the cardiovascular system. It is demonstrated to:

Raise levels of cholesterol.

Lessen your blood pressure.

Reduce your heart disease risk.

A major study commissioned by Swim England found that swimmers have a 41% lower risk of death due to heart disease or stroke than non-swimmers" and "a 28% lower risk of early death overall." Even cardiac rehabilitation patients can choose this option. Swimming can be tolerated by people recovering from heart failure or coronary artery disease, according to studies. Of course, if you are recovering from a major cardiac event or have a known medical condition, always consult your doctor before beginning a new exercise routine. Additionally, you should avoid swimming until your surgical incisions have healed if you have had open heart surgery or another procedure.

Strengthens your lungs

Swimming might be able to ease your breathing for you. It has been found to increase lung capacity and strength. If you've been diagnosed with asthma or chronic obstructive pulmonary disease (COPD), it can be a good exercise to try. Swimming "makes your body use oxygen more efficiently." Having said that, research has also shown that the disinfectants used to clean swimming pools can actually make asthma worse if you are exposed to them for a long time. Therefore, proceed with caution and always consult your doctor to ensure that swimming is safe for you.

HOW EXERCISES HELP YOU FROM AGING

Exercise is known to be useful for sound aging as it assists individuals with decreasing their gamble of persistent well-being conditions.1 Active exercise likewise affects body parts and cycles, for example,

Exercise plays a pivotal role in maintaining not just physical fitness but also in slowing down the aging process. As we age, our bodies undergo various physiological changes that can impact our overall health and quality of life. Regular exercise has been widely recognized as a powerful tool in promoting longevity and combating the effects of aging.

Exercise contributes significantly to maintaining muscle mass and strength, which naturally decline with age due to factors such as reduced protein synthesis and hormonal changes. Resistance training, in particular, helps stimulate muscle growth and counteracts sarcopenia, the age-related loss of muscle mass. By preserving muscle mass and strength, exercise supports mobility, balance, and independence in daily activities, thereby enhancing the overall quality of life for older adults

Cardiovascular exercise, such as jogging, swimming, or cycling, enhances heart and lung function. It improves circulation, lowers blood pressure, and increases aerobic capacity, all of which are vital for maintaining cardiovascular health as we age. Regular aerobic exercise also helps manage weight, reduce cholesterol levels, and improve glucose metabolism, thereby lowering the risk of chronic conditions such as heart disease, diabetes, and stroke.

Exercise promotes bone health and density, which tend to decline with age, leading to conditions like osteoporosis. Weight-bearing exercises like walking, dancing, and resistance training stimulate bone formation and strengthen bones, reducing the risk of fractures and maintaining skeletal integrity.

Beyond the physical benefits, exercise has profound effects on mental and cognitive health. Physical activity stimulates the release of endorphins, neurotransmitters that promote feelings of well-being and reduce stress and anxiety. Regular exercise has been shown to improve mood, alleviate symptoms of depression, and enhance cognitive function, including memory and learning ability. These cognitive benefits are particularly significant in aging populations, as exercise may help prevent or delay cognitive decline and neurodegenerative diseases such as Alzheimer's.

Exercise plays a crucial role in maintaining a healthy immune system, which tends to weaken with age. Physical activity enhances immune function by promoting circulation and lymphatic drainage, which helps the body fight off infections and illnesses more effectively.

To round it off, exercise is a potent anti-aging strategy that addresses multiple facets of health and well-being. By preserving muscle mass, enhancing cardiovascular function, improving bone density, boosting mental health, and supporting immune function, regular physical activity can significantly slow down the aging process and promote a longer, healthier life. Incorporating exercise into daily routines, regardless of age, is not just beneficial but essential for aging gracefully and maintaining overall vitality and independence.

CHAPTER THREE

ANTI-AGING DIETS

The impact of food on the aging process is profound and multifaceted, influencing not only our physical appearance but also our internal health and longevity. The choices we make in terms of diet can either accelerate or decelerate the aging process, making nutrition a critical factor in overall well-being.

To begin with, the foods we consume directly affect our skin, which is often one of the most visible indicators of aging. A diet high in sugar and refined carbohydrates can lead to glycation, a process where sugar molecules attach to proteins such as collagen and elastin in the skin. This can result in the formation of advanced glycation end-products (AGEs), which contribute to wrinkles, sagging skin, and loss of elasticity. Conversely, a diet rich in antioxidants, vitamins (such as vitamins C and E), and healthy fats can help protect the skin from oxidative stress and maintain its youthful appearance.

Beyond external appearance, dietary choices also impact internal aging processes. Chronic consumption of processed foods, high in trans fats, refined sugars, and excessive sodium, contributes to inflammation throughout the body. Inflammation is a key driver of aging and is associated with an increased risk of chronic diseases such as cardiovascular disease, diabetes, and arthritis. Conversely, a diet rich in anti-inflammatory foods such as fruits, vegetables, whole grains, fatty fish, nuts, and seeds can help reduce inflammation and support overall health.

The role of nutrition in maintaining cellular health and DNA integrity cannot be overstated. Certain nutrients, such as antioxidants (e.g., vitamins A, C, E, and selenium), phytochemicals (e.g., polyphenols), and omega-3 fatty acids, help protect cells from damage caused by free radicals and oxidative stress. Over time, cumulative damage to cellular DNA can contribute to cellular aging and increase the risk of mutations that may lead to cancer and other diseases.

Dietary habits play a crucial role in metabolic health and the regulation of hormone levels, both of which influence the aging process. Excessive consumption of calorie-dense, nutrient-poor foods can contribute to weight gain, insulin resistance, and metabolic syndrome, all of which are associated with accelerated aging and increased risk of chronic diseases. On the other hand, a balanced diet that includes adequate protein, healthy fats, and complex carbohydrates supports metabolic function and hormone balance, promoting overall health and longevity.

The impact of food on aging is intricate and far-reaching, affecting not only our external appearance but also our internal health and cellular function. Making informed dietary choices that prioritize nutrient density, antioxidant intake, and anti-inflammatory properties can significantly slow down the aging process and enhance overall well-being. By adopting a diet rich in whole foods, fruits, vegetables, lean proteins, and healthy fats while minimizing processed and sugary foods, individuals can support their body's natural mechanisms for repair, maintenance, and resilience against the aging effects of time.

Before we list the types of food that prevent us from aging. Here is a list of some foods that age us.

HERE ARE SOME FOOD THAT AGE US:
Processed meats
The processed meats sausage, hot dogs, pepperoni, and bacon are all examples of foods that can harm the skin. These meats contain a lot of sodium, saturated fats, and sulfite, all of which can make the skin dry out and weaken collagen by making inflammation worse. For economical protein choices, trade handled meats for eggs or beans.
Choose leaner meats like turkey and chicken if you want. Protein and amino acids that are

necessary for the natural production of collagen are abundant in these meats.

Alcohol

When it comes to the skin, alcohol can lead to a variety of issues, including wrinkles, loss of collagen, redness, and puffiness. Drinking alcohol reduces your intake of nutrients, hydration, and vitamin A, all of which contribute to wrinkle formation. Vitamin A plays a crucial role in the production of collagen and the growth of new cells, both of which contribute to elastic and wrinkle-free skin.

Coffee

Coffee contains the most caffeine, a naturally occurring substance in coffee beans, and added sugar is frequently found in on-the-go or homemade beverages. However, dehydration caused by these two ingredients can contribute to skin aging.

Dehydration can contribute to dry skin, which is one sign of aging skin. Sugar and caffeine should be avoided in order to prevent further dehydration; researchers have also discovered that caffeine can reduce the production of collagen, a protein that keeps skin firm and healthy, in human skin cells.

Fried Foods

Fried foods are another common source of AGEs and inflammation that can harm the skin. Increasing the temperature and conditions of cooking, such as frying, can double the amount of a marker for AGEs. Eat broiled food sources with some restraint. Try cooking the food in a different way if you can, like baking or mashing potatoes instead of French fries.

Sugary Drinks

Drinks with sugar and sweetness are obvious. Sweet and sugary drinks are bad because sugar and aging go hand in hand. Period. Your body's cells age more quickly the more you consume. These drinks have a lot of calories and sugar in them, and when combined with the bacteria in our mouth, they make acids that break down the enamel on our teeth and cause decay. Diabetes is at the top of the list of diseases that sugar consumption can cause, and the list goes on and on. Sugar consumption also has a clear effect on skin. It can start or exacerbate inflammation, clog pores, and worsen skin conditions like acne and eczema by increasing oil and sebum production.

Trans Fat

Trans fats can make your skin more vulnerable to sun damage, which is one of the most common causes of unfavorable aging signs like wrinkles and sagging skin. Considering them from a broader health perspective, numerous studies have shown that trans fats should be avoided because they raise bad cholesterol, which can result in a variety of unintended consequences, including diabetes, heart disease, stroke, and other chronic conditions.

White Flour

Refined grains are the basis for items like white bread, bagels, pretzels, pasta, and white bread. These foods lack the fiber and nutrients that make grains healthy in the first place. The foods become high-glycemic as a result of the milling process, which can cause rapid spikes in blood sugar and insulin levels. Oxidative stress and inflammation, which accelerate cellular aging, can be caused by this spike and subsequent drop in blood sugar. In addition, refined white flour, when compared to whole grains, lacks fiber and essential nutrients, depriving the body of key anti-aging nutrients like B vitamins, antioxidants, vitamin E, and minerals, further contributing to aging.

Cafe foods

Café food varieties, however advantageous, can add to maturing because of variables like elevated degrees of undesirable fats, including immersed and trans fats, prompting aggravation and a raised risk of age-related illnesses.

Additionally, even seemingly healthy restaurant fare can sneak in a lot of sugar, and most of these meals contain more sodium than a full day's worth. Meals from restaurants frequently contain a lot of salt and added sugar, which raises the risk of metabolic conditions like obesity and hypertension, which are linked to faster aging. Additionally, certain restaurant cooking techniques, such as frying or grilling at high temperatures, can result in the production of harmful compounds like AGEs and potentially carcinogenic substances, both of which contribute to cellular damage and accelerated aging.

On the contrary,

HERE ARE YOU THAT PREVENT YOU FROM AGING

Red bell pepper

Red bell peppers are stacked with antioxidants which rule with regards to aging well.

Notwithstanding their high level of L-ascorbic acid which is really great for collagen creation. Red bell peppers contain strong cell reinforcements called carotenoids. Carotenoids are plant shades answerable for the radiant red, yellow, and orange tones you see in many leafy foods. They have a number of anti-inflammatory properties, which can help your overall health and the health of your skin in particular.

Sweet potatoes

The antioxidant beta-carotene, which is converted into vitamin A and gives sweet potatoes their orange color, may assist in restoring skin elasticity and promoting cell turnover. This delicious root vegetable is a source of vitamins C and E, both of which may help protect our skin, despite the fact that it is considered a starchy vegetable.

Avocados

Avocados are the most tasty natural product we have with various supplements.

Avocados contain a lot of monounsaturated and polyunsaturated fats that can hydrate your skin and keep it from getting too dry. Additionally, it maintains proper immune system function by acting as an anti-inflammatory. The fruit's lutein and zeaxanthin may help shield your skin from UV damage, according to studies. It also has a lot of vitamins A, B, C, E, and K, all of which make your skin look and feel beautiful. Avocados can be added to salads or used to make healthy pudding.

Nuts

Proteins, vitamin E, minerals, essential oils, antioxidants, and other nutrients are abundant in nuts. Vitamin E, which helps shield the skin from the sun's ultraviolet rays, is abundant in almonds and walnuts. Vitamin E also makes your skin stronger and gives it a glow. For a little crunch, add some nuts to soup or sprinkle them on salads. Walnuts are high in omega-3 fats and have the highest antioxidant content of any nut. They are a great anti-inflammatory snack for better skin and overall health because of this combination. Pecans can likewise assist with working on your stomach-related well-being. Skin well-being is firmly connected to the soundness of our microbiome, and great stomach well-being assists the skin with keeping up with homeostasis for ideal insurance, temperature control, and liquid maintenance.

Vegetables

The majority of vegetables are high in nutrients and low in calories, making them excellent anti-aging foods. They incorporate cell reinforcements, which help in the counteraction of coronary illness, waterfalls, and certain malignancies. Carotenoids like lycopene and beta-carotene are found in a lot of vegetables. A diet high in carotenoids may protect the skin from the sun's UV rays, which are the leading cause of premature skin aging, according to some studies. Beta-carotene is abundant in pumpkin, sweet potatoes, and carrots, among other vegetables. Additionally, a potent antioxidant, vitamin C, is abundant in many vegetables. Collagen formation relies heavily on vitamin C. Although collagen is an essential component in the production of skin, its production begins to decline after the age of 25. The foods with the highest concentration of vitamin C include broccoli, bell peppers, tomatoes, and leafy greens. It's important to eat vegetables in a variety of colors because each color represents a different antioxidant that can help your skin and overall health. Always use sunscreen to protect your skin and aim for at least two servings of vegetables at each meal. Antioxidants, which can help your skin recover from sun damage and stay healthy, are abundant in vegetables.

Dark Chocolate

Chocolates are a great anti-aging food that also tastes great. Cancer prevention agents called polyphenols are viewed as bountiful in dull chocolate. Flavanols in it have been linked to a number of health benefits, including a lower risk of type 2 diabetes and heart disease. A diet rich in flavanols and other antioxidants is also thought to slow the aging process and protect the skin from solar damage.

When compared to the control group, participants in a high-quality 24-week trial who consumed cocoa beverages high in flavanols saw significant improvements in face wrinkles and skin elasticity.

Keep in mind that the proportion of cocoa is proportional to the flavanol level. The body uses flavanols in dark chocolate as antioxidants. It may help skin health.

Grapes

Resveratrol, which protects collagen from free radicals and keeps blood vessels healthy, is found in grapes. Collagen helps keep the skin's elasticity intact and keeps your skin looking young and radiant for a long time.

Tomatoes

In India, tomatoes have been added to the list of foods that fight wrinkles. Lycopene, a natural carotenoid that protects the skin from the sun, is abundant in them. Tomato juice can be consumed, but raw tomatoes can also be eaten, though cooked or processed tomatoes are preferable.

IMPACT OF EATING HEALTHY FOODS

Eating healthy foods has a profound impact on individuals and societies alike, influencing physical, mental, and even social well-being. This essay explores the multifaceted benefits of a balanced diet, ranging from personal health outcomes to broader societal implications.

The most immediate impact of consuming nutritious foods is on personal health. A diet rich in fruits, vegetables, whole grains, and lean proteins provides essential nutrients such as vitamins, minerals, and antioxidants. These nutrients support various bodily functions, including immune response, metabolism, and tissue repair. For instance, vitamin C from fruits helps boost immunity, while calcium from dairy products strengthens bones and teeth. Regular consumption of healthy fats, like those found in nuts and avocados, promotes heart health by lowering cholesterol levels. A balanced diet plays a crucial role in preventing chronic diseases. Obesity, diabetes, cardiovascular diseases, and certain cancers are often linked to poor dietary choices. By contrast, a diet low in processed foods and saturated fats, coupled with high fiber intake, can significantly reduce the risk of these ailments. For example, the Mediterranean diet, characterized by olive oil, fish, and vegetables, is renowned for its protective effects against heart diseases.

Going beyond physical health, eating well contributes to mental and emotional well-being. Studies indicate that certain nutrients influence brain function and mood regulation. Omega-3 fatty acids, prevalent in fish, walnuts, and flaxseeds, are associated with improved cognitive function and reduced risk of depression. Conversely, diets high in sugar and refined carbohydrates may contribute to mood swings and fatigue.

Eating good foods extends to economic and environmental dimensions.

Healthier populations incur lower healthcare costs and are more productive, benefiting economies. Sustainable food practices, such as organic farming and local produce sourcing, reduce environmental degradation and support biodiversity conservation. Thus, promoting healthy eating habits aligns with global efforts towards sustainable development goals.

The impact of eating healthy foods is profound and far-reaching. From enhancing personal health and well-being to fostering sustainable development, the benefits extend across individual, societal, and environmental realms. Embracing a balanced diet not only improves quality of life but also contributes to a healthier, more resilient society. As such, encouraging and facilitating access to nutritious foods should be a priority for governments, communities, and individuals alike in promoting long-term health and well-being.

CHAPTER FOUR

SLEEP AND REST

Sleep is an ordinary, reversible, repetitive condition of diminished responsiveness to outer excitement that is joined by mind-boggling and unsurprising changes in physiology. These changes include fluctuations in hormone levels, muscle relaxation, and coordinated, spontaneous, and internally generated brain activity. A concisely characterized explicit reason for rest stays indistinct, yet that is incomplete in light of the fact that rest is a powerful expression that impacts all physiology, as opposed to a singular organ or other separated actual framework. In contrast to wakefulness, which is characterized by a heightened potential for sensitivity and efficient responsiveness to external stimuli, sleep is characterized by sleepiness. The most striking manifestation of the more widespread phenomenon of periodicity in the activity or responsiveness of living tissue in higher vertebrates is the sleep-wakefulness alternation.

SLEEP AND ITS EFFECTS ON AGING

Aging is a complex process influenced by various factors, including genetics, lifestyle, and environmental conditions. Among these, sleep stands out as a crucial component impacting the aging process. Sleep affects numerous physiological and psychological aspects of human health, and its quality and duration play significant roles in how we age. This essay explores the multifaceted relationship between sleep and aging, examining how sleep influences cognitive function, physical health, emotional well-being, and overall longevity.

THE PHYSIOLOGY OF SLEEP

To understand the effects of sleep on aging, it is essential to comprehend the physiology of sleep itself. Sleep is a dynamic state characterized by a cyclical pattern of different stages. There are two main types of sleep: non-rapid eye movement (NREM) and rapid eye movement (REM) sleep.

NREM sleep is further divided into three stages, each representing a deeper level of sleep. Stage N1 is light sleep, Stage N2 is slightly deeper, and Stage N3, also known as slow-wave sleep (SWS), is the deepest form of sleep. REM sleep, on the other hand, is associated with vivid dreaming and significant brain activity.

During sleep, the body undergoes various restorative processes. For example, during NREM sleep, particularly in the SWS stage, the body repairs tissues, builds bone and muscle, and strengthens the immune system. REM sleep, in contrast, is critical for cognitive functions, such as memory consolidation, learning, and emotional regulation. A healthy sleep cycle, comprising all these stages, is essential for maintaining overall health and well-being.

COGNITIVE FUNCTION AND AGING

One of the most profound effects of sleep on aging is its impact on cognitive function. As people age, changes in sleep architecture are common. Older adults often experience less deep sleep (Stage N3) and more fragmented sleep patterns. These changes can have significant consequences for cognitive health.

Memory and Learning

Sleep, particularly REM sleep, plays a crucial role in memory consolidation and learning. During REM sleep, the brain processes and integrates new information, transferring it from short-term to long-term memory. Inadequate or disrupted sleep can impair these processes, leading to memory deficits. Studies have shown that older adults with poor sleep quality are more likely to experience cognitive decline and an increased risk of neurodegenerative diseases such as Alzheimer's disease.

Attention and Executive Function

Sleep is also vital for maintaining attention and executive function. Executive functions encompass higher-order cognitive processes, such as problem-solving, decision-making, and planning. Poor sleep can lead to reduced attention span, impaired decision-making, and decreased problem-solving abilities. These cognitive impairments can significantly impact daily functioning and quality of life in older adults.

PHYSICAL HEALTH AND AGING

The relationship between sleep and physical health is bidirectional. Poor sleep can contribute to various health problems, while certain health conditions can disrupt sleep. This interplay becomes particularly significant as individuals age.

Cardiovascular Health

Sleep is closely linked to cardiovascular health. During deep sleep, blood pressure drops, allowing the cardiovascular system to rest and recover. Chronic sleep deprivation or poor sleep quality can lead to hypertension (high blood pressure), a significant risk factor for cardiovascular diseases such as heart attacks and strokes. Older adults are already at an increased risk of cardiovascular issues, making adequate sleep even more crucial for maintaining heart health.

Metabolic Health

Sleep also plays a role in regulating metabolism. Disrupted sleep patterns can lead to metabolic disturbances, including insulin resistance and obesity. These metabolic issues are particularly concerning for older adults, as they can exacerbate the risk of developing type 2 diabetes and other age-related metabolic disorders. Additionally, poor sleep can affect appetite regulation, leading to unhealthy eating habits and weight gain.

Immune Function

The immune system relies on sleep to function optimally. During sleep, the body produces cytokines, proteins that help fight infection and inflammation. Chronic sleep deprivation can weaken the immune system, making individuals more susceptible to infections and illnesses. For older adults, who may already have a compromised immune system, good sleep is essential for maintaining immunity and overall health.

Musculoskeletal Health

Sleep is vital for musculoskeletal health. During deep sleep, the body repairs and builds bone and muscle tissues. Chronic sleep deprivation can impair these processes, leading to decreased bone density and muscle mass. This is particularly concerning for older adults, as they are already at an increased risk of osteoporosis and sarcopenia (age-related muscle loss). Adequate sleep can help mitigate these risks and promote better musculoskeletal health.

EMOTIONAL WELL-BEING AND AGING

Sleep has a profound impact on emotional well-being, and this relationship is particularly important as individuals age. Older adults often face various emotional challenges, such as increased stress, anxiety, and depression. Sleep can play a crucial role in managing these emotional states.

Stress and Anxiety

Poor sleep can exacerbate stress and anxiety levels. During sleep, the brain processes emotions and regulates stress hormones, such as cortisol. Chronic sleep deprivation can lead to dysregulation of these hormones, resulting in heightened stress and anxiety. Older adults with poor sleep quality may find it more challenging to cope with the stresses of aging, affecting their overall emotional well-being.

Depression

There is a well-established link between sleep disturbances and depression. Insomnia, a common sleep disorder, is both a symptom and a risk factor for depression. Older adults with chronic insomnia are more likely to develop depressive symptoms. Conversely, depression can also lead to sleep problems, creating a vicious cycle. Addressing sleep issues can be an essential component of managing depression in older adults.

Emotional Resilience

Adequate sleep is crucial for emotional resilience. It helps individuals regulate their emotions, respond better to stressors, and maintain a positive outlook on life. Older adults with good sleep quality are more likely to experience emotional stability and a higher quality of life.

SLEEP DISORDERS IN AGING

As individuals age, they are more likely to experience sleep disorders. These disorders can significantly impact their health and well-being.

Insomnia

Insomnia is one of the most common sleep disorders in older adults. It is characterized by difficulty falling asleep, staying asleep, or waking up too early. Chronic insomnia can lead to daytime fatigue, cognitive impairment, and emotional distress. Addressing insomnia is crucial for improving the overall quality of life in older adults.

Sleep Apnea

Sleep apnea is another prevalent sleep disorder among older adults. It is characterized by repeated interruptions in breathing during sleep, leading to fragmented sleep and reduced oxygen levels. Sleep apnea is associated with various health risks, including cardiovascular diseases, cognitive decline, and increased mortality. Proper diagnosis and treatment of sleep apnea can significantly improve sleep quality and overall health in older adults.

Restless Legs Syndrome (RLS)

RLS is a neurological disorder that causes uncomfortable sensations in the legs, leading to an irresistible urge to move them. This condition can disrupt sleep and lead to chronic sleep deprivation. RLS is more common in older adults and can significantly affect their sleep quality and daily functioning.

STRATEGIES FOR IMPROVING SLEEP IN OLDER ADULTS

Given the significant impact of sleep on aging, it is essential to implement strategies to improve sleep quality in older adults.

Sleep Hygiene

Practicing good sleep hygiene can help improve sleep quality. This includes maintaining a consistent sleep schedule, creating a comfortable sleep environment, and avoiding stimulants such as caffeine and alcohol close to bedtime. Engaging in relaxing activities before bed, such as reading or listening to calming music, can also promote better sleep.

Physical Activity

Regular physical activity can have a positive impact on sleep quality. Exercise helps regulate the sleep-wake cycle, reduces stress, and promotes overall physical health. However, it is essential to avoid vigorous exercise close to bedtime, as it can interfere with sleep.

Diet and Nutrition

A healthy diet can contribute to better sleep. Avoiding heavy meals and excessive fluid intake close to bedtime can prevent discomfort and frequent trips to the bathroom during the night. Additionally, certain foods, such as those rich in tryptophan (an amino acid that promotes sleep), can help improve sleep quality.

Cognitive Behavioral Therapy for Insomnia (CBT-I)

CBT-I is a structured program that helps individuals identify and change negative thoughts and behaviors related to sleep. It is an effective treatment for chronic insomnia and can significantly improve sleep quality in older adults.

Medical Interventions

In some cases, medical interventions may be necessary to address sleep disorders. This can include medications, such as sleep aids or treatments for underlying conditions like sleep apnea. It is essential for older adults to consult healthcare professionals to determine the most appropriate treatment options

BENEFITS OF SLEEP AND REST

Sleep is a fundamental aspect of human life that is often undervalued in today's fast-paced society. While many people prioritize work, social activities, and digital engagements over rest, understanding the myriad benefits of sleep is essential for fostering a healthy lifestyle.

PHYSICAL HEALTH BENEFITS

Immune Function

Sleep plays a crucial role in maintaining a strong immune system. During sleep, the body produces cytokines, proteins that help combat infection and inflammation. A lack of sleep can decrease the production of these protective substances, making individuals more susceptible to illnesses. Studies show that people who do not get adequate sleep are more likely to catch colds and other infections.

Weight Management

Quality sleep is linked to weight regulation. Sleep deprivation can disrupt the balance of hormones that regulate appetite, leading to increased cravings and unhealthy eating patterns. The hormones ghrelin (which stimulates appetite) and leptin (which signals satiety) are adversely affected by lack of sleep. As a result, individuals may experience weight gain and obesity-related health issues.

Cardiovascular Health

Sleep is vital for heart health. Research indicates that inadequate sleep is associated with increased risks of heart disease, hypertension, and stroke. During deep sleep, the body undergoes processes that help lower blood pressure and reduce stress on the heart, contributing to cardiovascular health and longevity.

MENTAL WELL-BEING

Stress Reduction

Sleep acts as a natural stress reliever. Adequate rest helps regulate mood and manage stress levels, which can have a direct impact on mental health. Insufficient sleep can lead to increased levels of cortisol, the body's primary stress hormone, exacerbating feelings of anxiety and depression. Prioritizing sleep can lead to improved emotional stability and resilience.

Mental Clarity and Emotional Balance

Quality sleep contributes to better emotional regulation. It helps individuals process experiences and emotions, allowing for clearer thinking and improved decision-making. Studies have shown that those who sleep well are better equipped to handle emotional challenges and exhibit greater empathy and social awareness.

COGNITIVE PERFORMANCE

Memory Consolidation

One of the most significant benefits of sleep is its role in memory consolidation. During sleep, particularly during the REM (Rapid Eye Movement) phase, the brain processes and organizes information gathered throughout the day. This process strengthens neural connections, enhancing learning and retention. Consequently, individuals who prioritize sleep often perform better academically and professionally.

Enhanced Concentration and Productivity

Sleep is essential for cognitive functions such as attention, problem-solving, and creativity. A well-rested brain can focus more effectively, leading to increased productivity and efficiency in daily tasks. Conversely, lack of sleep impairs cognitive performance, making it difficult to concentrate and increasing the likelihood of mistakes.

IMPACT ON LONGEVITY AND QUALITY OF LIFE

Improved Life Satisfaction

A regular sleep schedule and adequate rest contribute to overall life satisfaction. Individuals who sleep well tend to report higher levels of happiness and fulfillment in their personal and professional lives. Sleep enhances interpersonal relationships and social interactions, as well-rested individuals are generally more engaged and positive.

Longevity

Research indicates a strong correlation between sleep duration and longevity. Studies suggest that individuals who consistently get 7-9 hours of sleep per night have a lower risk of premature death compared to those who experience sleep deprivation. Adequate sleep contributes to overall health, reducing the risk of chronic illnesses that can impact lifespan.

TIPS FOR IMPROVING SLEEP QUALITY

To reap the numerous benefits of sleep, it is essential to establish healthy sleep habits. Here are some strategies to enhance sleep quality:

Establish a Sleep Schedule

Go to bed and wake up at the same time every day to regulate your body's internal clock.

Create a Restful Environment

Ensure your sleeping area is dark, quiet, and cool to promote relaxation.

Limit Screen Time

Reduce exposure to screens at least an hour before bedtime, as blue light can interfere with the production of melatonin, the sleep hormone.

Practice Relaxation Techniques

Engage in relaxation practices such as meditation, deep breathing, or gentle yoga before bedtime to calm the mind.

Be Mindful of Diet:

 Avoid heavy meals, caffeine, and alcohol close to bedtime, as they can disrupt sleep patterns.

Stay Active

Regular physical activity can promote better sleep, but try to avoid vigorous exercise close to bedtime.

The benefits of sleep extend far beyond mere rest. From enhancing physical health to improving mental well-being and cognitive performance, sleep is a vital component of a healthy lifestyle. In our busy world, prioritizing sleep is essential for overall health, longevity, and happiness. By understanding the significance of sleep and adopting healthy sleep habits, individuals can unlock the full potential of this natural restorative process, leading to a more balanced and fulfilling life. Making sleep a priority is not just a personal choice; it is an investment in one's health and future well-being. Conclusively, sleep plays a vital role in the aging process, influencing cognitive function, physical health, emotional well-being, and overall longevity. As individuals age, changes in sleep patterns and an increased prevalence of sleep disorders can pose significant challenges to maintaining good health. Understanding the intricate relationship between sleep and aging is crucial for developing effective strategies to improve sleep quality and promote healthy aging.

By prioritizing sleep hygiene, engaging in regular physical activity, maintaining a healthy diet, and seeking appropriate medical interventions when necessary, older adults can enhance their sleep quality and overall well-being. Addressing sleep issues is not only essential for improving the quality of life in older adults but also for promoting healthy aging and reducing the risk of age-related health problems. Ultimately, ensuring adequate and restful sleep is a key component of aging gracefully and maintaining vitality throughout the lifespan.

CHAPTER FIVE

STRESS AND AGING

Stress is a characteristic human response that happens to everybody. In point of fact, your body is made to feel and respond to stress. At the point when you experience changes or difficulties (stressors), your body produces physical and mental reactions.

Your body can better adapt to new situations by responding to stress. Positive stress can keep you alert, motivated, and prepared to avoid danger. A stress response, for instance, may encourage your body to work harder and stay awake for longer if you have an important test coming up. However, when stressors persist without relief or periods of relaxation, stress becomes a problem.

HARMFUL EFFECTS OF STRESS ON AGING

Stress is a ubiquitous part of modern life, and its impact on health and well-being is profound.

While occasional stress can serve as a motivator or a response to immediate threats, chronic stress can have deleterious effects on the body and mind. Among its various impacts, stress plays a significant role in the aging process, accelerating biological aging and increasing the risk of age-related diseases. This essay explores the harmful effects of stress on aging, examining how chronic stress influences physical health, cognitive function, emotional well-being, and overall longevity.

Physical Health and Aging

One of the primary ways stress affects aging is through its impact on physical health. Chronic stress triggers a cascade of physiological responses that can accelerate the aging process and contribute to various health problems.

Cardiovascular Health:

Chronic stress stimulates the release of stress hormones such as cortisol and adrenaline, which prepare the body for a "fight-or-flight" response. While this response is useful in acute situations, prolonged exposure to these hormones can lead to hypertension (high blood pressure), increased heart rate, and inflammation. These changes place extra strain on the cardiovascular system, increasing the risk of heart disease, stroke, and other cardiovascular conditions. Research has shown that individuals with high levels of stress are more likely to develop atherosclerosis (hardening of the arteries), a major risk factor for heart attacks and strokes.

Immune System:

Stress also affects the immune system, impairing its ability to function properly. Chronic stress suppresses immune responses, making the body more susceptible to infections and diseases. This weakened immune function is particularly concerning for older adults, who are already at a higher risk of infections due to age-related immune decline. Additionally, chronic stress can promote chronic inflammation, which is associated with various age-related diseases, including arthritis, diabetes, and certain cancers.

Cellular Aging:

At the cellular level, stress can accelerate aging through the shortening of telomeres, the protective caps at the ends of chromosomes. Telomeres naturally shorten with age, but chronic stress can hasten this process. Shortened telomeres are associated with a higher risk of age-related diseases and reduced lifespan. Studies have shown that individuals exposed to chronic stress, such as caregivers of chronically ill patients, tend to have shorter telomeres compared to those with lower stress levels.

Cognitive Function and Stress

The impact of stress on cognitive function is another significant factor in the aging process. Chronic stress can lead to cognitive decline and increase the risk of neurodegenerative diseases.

Memory and Learning:

Stress affects the hippocampus, a region of the brain critical for memory and learning. Elevated levels of cortisol can damage hippocampal neurons, leading to impaired memory and cognitive function. Older adults with chronic stress are more likely to experience memory problems and are at a higher risk of developing conditions such as Alzheimer's disease.

Attention and Executive Function:

Chronic stress can impair attention and executive function, which includes higher-order cognitive processes such as problem-solving, decision-making, and planning. These cognitive impairments can affect daily functioning and quality of life. For instance, older adults under chronic stress may struggle with tasks that require sustained attention or complex decision-making.

Emotional Well-Being and Stress

Stress has a profound impact on emotional well-being, and its effects can be particularly detrimental as individuals age. Chronic stress can exacerbate emotional challenges and contribute to mental health issues.

Depression and Anxiety:

Chronic stress is a significant risk factor for depression and anxiety. Prolonged exposure to stress hormones can alter brain chemistry, leading to mood disorders. Older adults with chronic stress are more likely to develop depressive symptoms and anxiety, which can further affect their physical health and quality of life.

Emotional Resilience

Stress can erode emotional resilience, making it harder for individuals to cope with life's challenges. This is particularly important for older adults, who may face various stressors such as retirement, loss of loved ones, and health issues. Reduced emotional resilience can lead to increased vulnerability to stress and a lower overall sense of well-being.

Overall Longevity

The cumulative effects of chronic stress on physical health, cognitive function, and emotional well-being can ultimately impact overall longevity. Studies have shown that individuals with high levels of chronic stress tend to have shorter lifespans compared to those with lower stress levels. Chronic stress accelerates the aging process, increasing the risk of age-related diseases and reducing the overall quality of life.

Chronic stress has significant harmful effects on the aging process, impacting physical health, cognitive function, emotional well-being, and overall longevity. By understanding the mechanisms through which stress accelerates aging and implementing strategies to manage stress, individuals can promote healthier aging and improve their quality of life. Addressing chronic stress is essential for reducing the risk of age-related diseases, enhancing cognitive function, and maintaining emotional well-being throughout the aging process.

TIPS FOR MANAGING STRESS

Managing stress is crucial for maintaining overall health and well-being. Chronic stress can lead to a variety of physical and mental health issues, including anxiety, depression, heart disease, and weakened immune function. By incorporating effective stress management techniques into your daily routine, you can reduce the negative impact of stress and improve your quality of life. Here are some practical tips for managing stress:

Exercise Regularly

Physical activity is one of the most effective ways to combat stress. Exercise releases endorphins, which are natural mood lifters. It also helps reduce the levels of stress hormones like cortisol. Aim for at least 30 minutes of moderate exercise most days of the week. Activities such as walking, jogging, swimming, cycling, and yoga can be particularly beneficial. Even short bouts of physical activity, like taking a brisk walk, can help reduce stress.

Practice Mindfulness and Meditation

Mindfulness and meditation techniques can significantly reduce stress levels. Mindfulness involves focusing on the present moment and accepting it without judgment. Meditation practices, such as deep breathing exercises, progressive muscle relaxation, and guided imagery, can help calm the mind and reduce stress. Even spending a few minutes each day in meditation can make a big difference.

Maintain a Healthy Diet

What you eat can affect your stress levels. A balanced diet rich in fruits, vegetables, whole grains, lean proteins, and healthy fats can help your body cope with stress more effectively. Avoid excessive caffeine and sugar, which can increase anxiety and stress. Staying hydrated by drinking plenty of water is also essential for maintaining energy levels and reducing stress.

Get Enough Sleep

Adequate sleep is crucial for managing stress. Lack of sleep can make it harder to cope with stress and can lead to irritability and exhaustion. Aim for 7-9 hours of quality sleep each night. Establish a regular sleep routine by going to bed and waking up at the same time each day. Create a relaxing bedtime routine, avoid screens before bed, and make your sleep environment comfortable and conducive to rest.

Stay Connected

Social support is vital for managing stress. Spending time with friends and family can provide emotional support and help you feel more connected and understood. Talking about your feelings with someone you trust can also provide relief. Joining clubs and groups or engaging in community activities can help you build a supportive social network.

Learn to Say No

Overcommitting yourself can lead to increased stress. Learning to say no to additional responsibilities or demands on your time is essential for maintaining balance and preventing burnout. Prioritize your tasks and focus on what is most important. Delegate tasks when possible and set realistic goals for yourself.

Practice Time Management

Effective time management can help reduce stress by allowing you to feel more in control of your day. Create a daily schedule, prioritize your tasks, and break larger tasks into smaller, manageable steps. Avoid procrastination by setting deadlines and tackling high-priority tasks first.

Engage in Hobbies and Interests

Participating in activities you enjoy can be a great way to relieve stress. Hobbies and interests provide a break from daily pressures and allow you to focus on something pleasurable. Whether it's reading, gardening, painting, playing a musical instrument, or any other activity, make time for the things you love.

Seek Professional Help

If stress becomes overwhelming, seeking professional help from a therapist or counselor can be beneficial. Cognitive-behavioral therapy (CBT) and other therapeutic approaches can provide you with tools and strategies to manage stress more effectively. Don't hesitate to reach out for help if you need it.

Managing stress is an essential aspect of maintaining a healthy and balanced life. By incorporating regular exercise, mindfulness practices, a healthy diet, adequate sleep, social support, and effective time management into your routine, you can reduce stress levels and enhance your overall well-being. Remember that it's important to find what works best for you and to make stress management a priority in your life.

CHAPTER SIX

AGING GRACEFULLY

Aging is a natural and inevitable part of life. While it brings wisdom and experience, it can also present challenges, both physically and emotionally. Aging gracefully involves embracing the aging process with a positive mindset and making lifestyle choices that promote overall health and well-being. This essay explores the multifaceted approach to aging gracefully, focusing on physical health, mental well-being, social connections, and a positive outlook on life.

Physical health is a cornerstone of aging gracefully. As we age, our bodies undergo numerous changes, including a decrease in muscle mass, bone density, and metabolic rate. To counter these changes, it is essential to maintain an active lifestyle. Regular exercise not only helps keep the body strong and flexible but also enhances mental health by releasing endorphins, which are natural mood lifters. Engaging in activities such as walking, swimming, yoga, or strength training can improve cardiovascular health, increase muscle strength, and enhance balance and coordination.

Nutrition also plays a crucial role in aging gracefully. A balanced diet rich in fruits, vegetables, whole grains, lean proteins, and healthy fats provides the necessary nutrients to support overall health. Antioxidant-rich foods, such as berries, nuts, and green leafy vegetables, help combat oxidative stress, which contributes to the aging process. Staying hydrated by drinking plenty of water is equally important, as it helps maintain skin elasticity and supports various bodily functions.

Regular medical check-ups are vital for early detection and management of age-related health issues. Preventive care, such as vaccinations, screenings for chronic conditions, and regular dental visits, can help maintain good health and prevent complications. Listening to your body and addressing any health concerns promptly is essential for aging gracefully. Remember to stay safe.

Cultivating Mental Well-Being
Mental well-being is another critical aspect of aging gracefully. Cognitive decline is a common concern as we age, but there are several ways to keep the mind sharp and engaged. Lifelong learning and mental stimulation can help maintain cognitive function. Engaging in activities that challenge the brain, such as puzzles, reading, learning a new language, or playing musical instruments, can enhance mental agility and memory.

Stress management is also crucial for mental well-being. Chronic stress can take a toll on both physical and mental health, accelerating the aging process. Techniques such as mindfulness meditation, deep breathing exercises, and yoga can help reduce stress and promote relaxation. Regular physical activity, as mentioned earlier, also contributes to stress reduction and overall mental well-being.

Quality sleep is essential for cognitive function and emotional resilience. As we age, changes in sleep patterns are common, but maintaining good sleep hygiene can improve sleep quality. Creating a relaxing bedtime routine, avoiding screens before bed, and ensuring a comfortable sleep environment can promote restful sleep. Addressing sleep disorders, such as insomnia or sleep apnea, with the help of healthcare professionals is also important for maintaining mental well-being. It's very important to get good sleep.

Fostering Social Connections
Social connections are vital for emotional health and aging gracefully. Maintaining strong relationships with family, friends, and community members provides emotional support and a sense of belonging. Social interactions can boost mood, reduce feelings of loneliness, and enhance overall life satisfaction. Participating in

social activities, such as clubs, volunteer work, or group exercises, can help foster new friendships and strengthen existing ones.

Having a strong support network is particularly important during challenging times, such as dealing with loss or health issues. Sharing experiences and emotions with others can provide comfort and reduce the burden of stress. Additionally, intergenerational relationships, such as spending time with younger family members or mentoring, can bring joy and a sense of purpose.

Adopting a Positive Outlook
A positive outlook on life is a key component of aging gracefully. Embracing the aging process with acceptance and optimism can significantly impact overall well-being. Instead of focusing on the limitations that come with age, it is beneficial to appreciate the wisdom and experiences gained over the years. Cultivating gratitude and practicing mindfulness can help

shift the focus from what is lost to what is still achievable and enjoyable.

Having a sense of purpose and staying engaged in meaningful activities can enhance life satisfaction. Pursuing hobbies, volunteering, or taking up new interests can provide a sense of accomplishment and fulfillment. Setting realistic goals and celebrating small achievements can also boost self-esteem and motivation.

Resilience is an important trait for aging gracefully. Life is full of ups and downs, and the ability to adapt to changes and bounce back from adversity is crucial for maintaining a positive outlook. Building resilience involves developing coping strategies, seeking support when needed, and maintaining a flexible attitude toward life's challenges.

The Role of Self-Care
Self-care is an essential practice for aging gracefully. Taking time to care for oneself physically, mentally, and emotionally can

improve quality of life and overall well-being. Self-care practices can vary widely and should be tailored to individual preferences and needs.

Physical self-care includes activities that promote physical health, such as regular exercise, balanced nutrition, and adequate sleep. It also involves listening to the body and addressing any health concerns promptly. Engaging in activities that promote relaxation and reduce stress, such as taking a warm bath, getting a massage, or spending time in nature, can also be beneficial.

Mental and emotional self-care involves practices that nurture the mind and emotions. This can include engaging in hobbies, practicing mindfulness, seeking therapy or counseling, and connecting with loved ones. Setting boundaries and learning to say no to additional stressors can also be an important aspect of self-care.

Embracing Change and Flexibility

Aging gracefully involves embracing change and maintaining flexibility. Life is full of transitions, and being able to adapt to new circumstances is crucial for maintaining well-being. This can include changes in physical abilities, relationships, or living situations. Developing a flexible mindset and being open to new experiences can help navigate these changes more smoothly.

Planning for the future can also reduce stress and increase a sense of control. This can include financial planning, discussing healthcare preferences, and making legal arrangements, such as creating a will or advanced directives. Having a plan in place can provide peace of mind and allow for more focus on enjoying life.

The Importance of Lifelong Learning

Lifelong learning is an important component of aging gracefully. Engaging in continuous learning can keep the mind sharp, enhance cognitive function, and provide a sense of purpose and fulfillment. This can include formal education, such as taking classes or pursuing degrees, or informal learning, such as reading, attending lectures, or learning new skills.

Staying curious and open to new experiences can lead to personal growth and new opportunities. Lifelong learning can also foster social connections by providing opportunities to meet new people and engage in shared interests. Embracing a growth mindset, where challenges are viewed as opportunities for learning and development, can contribute to overall well-being and life satisfaction.

Aging gracefully is a holistic approach that involves embracing physical health, mental well-being, social connections, a positive outlook, self-care, flexibility, and lifelong learning. By adopting healthy lifestyle choices, managing stress, fostering strong relationships, and maintaining a positive attitude, individuals can enhance their quality of life and well-being as they age. Embracing the aging process with acceptance and optimism can lead to a more fulfilling and meaningful life, where the focus is on enjoying each moment and appreciating the wisdom and experiences gained over the years. Aging gracefully is about living life to the fullest, regardless of age, and finding joy and purpose in every stage of life.

CONCLUSION

The quest to avoid aging is a pursuit that has captivated humanity for centuries, deeply rooted in our desire for longevity, vitality, and the perpetuation of youth. Throughout "outlive your longevity" we have explored a myriad of strategies, both ancient and contemporary, aimed at decelerating the aging process and enhancing our quality of life. As we reach the conclusion of this journey, it is essential to synthesize the knowledge and insights gained and to understand that while aging is an inevitable biological process, there are numerous ways to influence how gracefully and healthily we experience it.

Embracing a Holistic Approach
One of the central themes of this book is the importance of a holistic approach to aging. Aging is not merely a physical phenomenon but

a multifaceted process that encompasses physical health, mental well-being, emotional balance, and social connections. By addressing all these aspects, we can create a comprehensive strategy that promotes longevity and vitality.

Not to forget, physically, maintaining an active lifestyle, consuming a balanced diet, and getting adequate rest are fundamental. Regular exercise strengthens muscles, improves cardiovascular health, and boosts mental health. A diet rich in antioxidants, vitamins, and minerals supports bodily functions and combats oxidative stress, a key contributor to aging. Adequate sleep allows the body to repair and rejuvenate, while also supporting cognitive function and emotional health.

Mentally, engaging in lifelong learning, challenging the brain with new activities, and practicing mindfulness can keep the mind sharp and resilient. Mental stimulation, whether through reading, puzzles, or social interactions, helps maintain cognitive functions and may delay the onset of age-related cognitive decline.

Emotionally, managing stress through techniques such as meditation, yoga, and deep breathing exercises is crucial. Chronic stress accelerates aging by increasing the levels of cortisol, a hormone that can harm various bodily systems over time. Cultivating emotional resilience and maintaining a positive outlook can significantly impact how we age.

On a social point of view, strong relationships and a sense of community provide emotional support and contribute to a longer, healthier life. Social interactions combat feelings of loneliness and depression, which are common in older age and can negatively affect overall health.

The Role of Modern Science and Medicine

The advancements in science and medicine have revolutionized our understanding of aging and provided new tools to combat its effects. Throughout this book, we have delved into the latest research and techniques that hold promise in the fight against aging.

Genetics plays a crucial role in how we age, and modern science has begun to unlock the secrets of our DNA. Research into telomeres, the protective caps at the ends of chromosomes, has shown that their length correlates with aging and health. Interventions that maintain telomere length, such as specific dietary components, exercise, and stress reduction, are being explored as potential anti-aging strategies.

Breakthroughs in biotechnology and also regenerative medicine offer exciting possibilities. Stem cell therapy, which aims to repair or replace damaged tissues, holds promise for treating age-related diseases and extending healthy lifespan. Similarly, advancements in gene editing techniques like CRISPR could one day allow us to correct genetic mutations associated with aging and age-related conditions. Pharmaceutical developments, including the exploration of senolytics (drugs that target and eliminate senescent cells), offer another avenue for combating aging. Senescent cells, often referred to as "zombie cells," accumulate with age and contribute to inflammation and tissue deterioration. Removing these cells has shown promise in extending health span in animal studies, and human trials are underway.

The Power of Prevention

Prevention is a recurring theme in the quest to avoid aging. Many of the strategies discussed in this book emphasize the importance of proactive measures to maintain health and prevent age-related decline.

Preventive healthcare, including regular check-ups, screenings, and vaccinations, is vital. Early detection of conditions such as hypertension, diabetes, and cancer can lead to more effective treatment and better outcomes. Preventive measures also include lifestyle choices such as avoiding smoking, limiting alcohol consumption, and protecting skin from excessive sun exposure to reduce the risk of chronic diseases and maintain overall health.

Nutrition, likewise plays a pivotal role in prevention. Adopting a diet rich in fruits, vegetables, whole grains, lean proteins, and healthy fats can prevent many chronic diseases associated with aging. Specific nutrients, such as omega-3 fatty acids, antioxidants, and vitamins, have been shown to support brain health, reduce inflammation, and protect against cellular damage.

Physical activity is another cornerstone of preventive health. Regular exercise not only helps maintain a healthy weight and strengthens muscles and bones but also reduces the risk of cardiovascular diseases, diabetes, and certain cancers. It also enhances mental health by reducing symptoms of depression and anxiety.

The Influence of Mindset and Attitude
The mind-body connection is a powerful factor in aging, and our mindset and attitude toward aging can significantly influence how we experience it. Throughout this book, we have explored the impact of psychological factors on aging and how cultivating a positive outlook can lead to a more fulfilling and healthy life.

A growth mindset, which embraces challenges and views failures as opportunities for learning, can enhance resilience and adaptability. This mindset fosters continuous personal growth and helps individuals navigate the changes and uncertainties that come with aging.

Gratitude is another powerful tool. Practicing gratitude shifts focus from what is lacking to what is present and valuable. This positive shift in perspective can improve emotional well-being and reduce stress, contributing to overall health.

Mindfulness and meditation practices have been shown to reduce stress, improve mental clarity, and enhance emotional regulation. These practices encourage living in the present moment and accepting it without judgment, which can reduce anxiety about aging and future uncertainties.

The Importance of Purpose and Engagement
Having a sense of purpose and staying engaged in meaningful activities is crucial for aging well. Throughout this book, we have highlighted the importance of finding and pursuing passions,

hobbies, and interests that bring joy and fulfillment.

Purpose provides a reason to get up in the morning and can significantly impact mental and physical health. Studies have shown that individuals with a strong sense of purpose tend to live longer, healthier lives. Purpose can be found in various forms, whether through career, volunteer work, creative pursuits, or relationships.

Staying engaged in social and community activities fosters a sense of belonging and connection. Volunteering, participating in clubs or groups, and maintaining social relationships can enhance life satisfaction and combat feelings of loneliness and isolation.

Embracing Aging with Acceptance

While the title "Outlive your longevity" suggests a desire to halt the aging process, it is important to recognize that aging is an intrinsic part of the human experience. Acceptance of this reality does not equate to resignation; rather, it means embracing aging with grace and dignity.

Acceptance involves recognizing the changes that come with aging and adapting to them with a positive attitude. It means valuing the wisdom and experiences that come with age and appreciating the journey rather than fixating solely on the destination.

This book encourages a balanced perspective on aging—one that seeks to optimize health and well-being while acknowledging and respecting the natural course of life. By embracing aging with acceptance, we can focus on making the most of each stage of life and finding joy in the present moment.

The Interconnectedness of Strategies

The strategies discussed in this book are interconnected and mutually reinforcing. Physical health supports mental well-being, and vice versa. Social connections enhance emotional health, which in turn supports physical health. Preventive measures and a positive mindset create a foundation for healthy aging.

For instance, regular exercise not only strengthens the body but also boosts mood and cognitive function. A balanced diet supports physical health and reduces the risk of chronic diseases, while also providing the energy needed to stay active and engaged. Social interactions provide emotional support and mental stimulation, contributing to overall well-being.

By integrating these strategies into our daily lives, we create a synergistic effect that promotes healthy aging. It is not about finding a single solution but rather about adopting a comprehensive approach that addresses all aspects of our being.

Moving Forward

As we conclude "Outlive your longevity," it is clear that while we cannot stop the passage of time, we have the power to influence how we age. The knowledge and strategies shared in this book provide a roadmap for aging gracefully, healthily, and joyfully.

The journey to avoid aging is not about seeking immortality but about maximizing the quality of life and making the most of each moment. It is about embracing the changes that come with age and finding ways to thrive at every stage.

Moving forward, let us carry with us the wisdom and insights gained from this exploration. Let us commit to making choices that support our health and well-being, nurturing our bodies, minds, and spirits. Let us cherish our relationships, cultivate a positive outlook, and engage in meaningful activities that bring joy and fulfillment.

In the end, the true essence of avoiding aging lies not in defying the natural process but in living fully and vibrantly, regardless of the number of years we have lived. It is about celebrating life, embracing change, and finding beauty and purpose in every phase of our journey. May we all age with grace, wisdom, and a boundless zest for life.